# DEPARTMENT CHAIR

## Essentials Handbook

Richard A. Sheff, MD

Robert J. Marder, MD

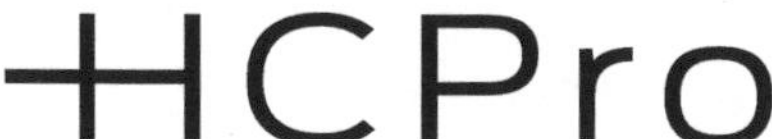

*Department Chair Essentials Handbook* is published by HCPro, Inc.

 5 4 3 2 1

ISBN: 978-1-60146-946-5



Richard A. Sheff, MD, Author
Robert J. Marder, MD, Author
Katrina Gravel, Editorial Assistant
Matt Sharpe, Production Supervisor
Elizabeth Jones, Editor
Erin Callahan, Associate Editorial Director
Shane Katz, Art Director
Jean St. Pierre, Senior Director of Operations



Arrangements can be made for quantity discounts. For more information, contact:

HCPro, Inc.
75 Sylvan Street, Suite A-101
Danvers, MA 01923
Telephone: 800-650-6787 or 781-639-1872
Fax: 800-639-8511
Email: *customerservice@hcpro.com*

**Visit HCPro online at: *www.hcpro.com* and *www.hcmarketplace.com***

07/2012
21975

# Contents



  

# Figure List



  

# About the Authors

## Richard A. Sheff, MD

**Richard A. Sheff, MD,** is principal and chief medical officer with The Greeley Company, a division of HCPro, Inc., in Danvers, Mass. He brings more than 25 years of healthcare management and leadership experience to his work with physicians, hospitals, and healthcare systems across the country. With his distinctive combination of medical, healthcare, and management acumen, Dr. Sheff develops tailored solutions to the unique needs of physicians and hospitals. He consults, authors, and presents on a wide range of healthcare management and leadership issues, including governance, physician-hospital alignment, medical staff leadership development, ED call, peer review, hospital performance improvement, disruptive physician management, conflict resolution, physician employment and contracting, healthcare systems, service line management, hospitalist program optimization, patient safety and error reduction, credentialing, strategic planning, regulatory compliance, and helping physicians rediscover the joy of medicine.

  

## Robert J. Marder, MD

**Robert J. Marder, MD,** is an advisory consultant and director of medical staff services with The Greeley Company, a division of HCPro, Inc., in Danvers, Mass. He brings more than 25 years of healthcare leadership and management experience to his work with physicians, hospitals, and healthcare organizations across the country. Dr. Marder's many roles in senior hospital medical administration and operations management in academic and community hospital settings make him uniquely qualified to assist physicians and hospitals in developing solutions for complex medical staff and hospital performance issues. He consults, authors, and presents on a wide range of healthcare leadership issues, including effective and efficient peer review, physician performance measurement and improvement, hospital quality measurement systems and performance improvement, patient safety/error reduction, and utilization management.

# DOWNLOAD YOUR MATERIALS NOW

This handbook includes a customizable presentation that organizations can use to train physician leaders. The presentation complements the information provided in this handbook and can be downloaded at the following link:

www.hcpro.com/downloads/10553

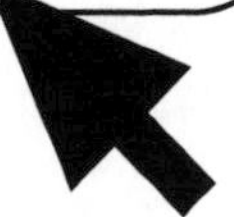

**Thank you for purchasing this product!**

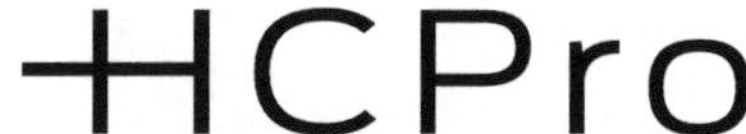

CHAPTER 1

# Roles and Responsibilities of the Department Chair

This orientation handbook is intended to provide both new and experienced department chairs with the tools needed to understand and carry out the responsibilities of a medical staff department chair. This training will arm department leaders with the information, knowledge, and skills that they may not have learned in medical school or residency training, but that are critical when serving in this leadership role.

## Board, Administration, and Medical Staff Relationships

The first step in understanding your responsibilities as department chair is understanding your role in relation to the rest of your organization. Figure 1.1 is an organizational chart that depicts the relationship between the board, administration, and medical staff.

Figure 1.1

**BOARD, ADMINISTRATION, AND MEDICAL STAFF STRUCTURE**

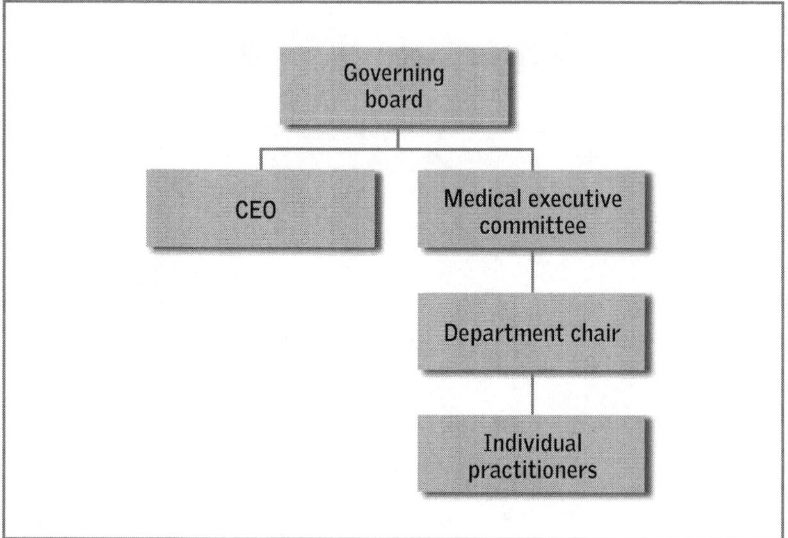


As you can see in Figure 1.1, the organizational chart begins with a governing board. The governing board hires a CEO, who hires vice presidents, who hire directors, and so on. The governing board assigns responsibilities to management and holds them accountable by holding the CEO accountable. The governing board also assigns responsibilities to the medical staff.

Keep in mind that the medical executive committee (MEC) primarily serves as the senior governing entity within the medical staff. Although the full medical staff has certain reserved powers through elected officers and bylaw amendments, the MEC is primarily responsible for coordinating and managing most of the work of the medical staff. With this in mind, department chairs must understand that they are accountable to the MEC.

  

Individual practitioners within a specific department are accountable to the department chair, who is accountable to the MEC, which in turn is accountable to the governing board. Although the department chair certainly has a role in advocating for members of his or her department, he or she also has the responsibility to fulfill the functions of the medical staff as delegated to the department chair by the MEC.

The department chair has the challenging task of recognizing where he or she fits within the hierarchy of the traditional medical staff organization while acknowledging his or her role as an advocate for the medical staff. Department chairs should not be subservient to the board. We refer to this balancing act as the three-legged stool model. See Figure 1.2 below.

Figure 1.2 **BOARD, ADMINISTRATION, AND MEDICAL STAFF RELATIONSHIPS**

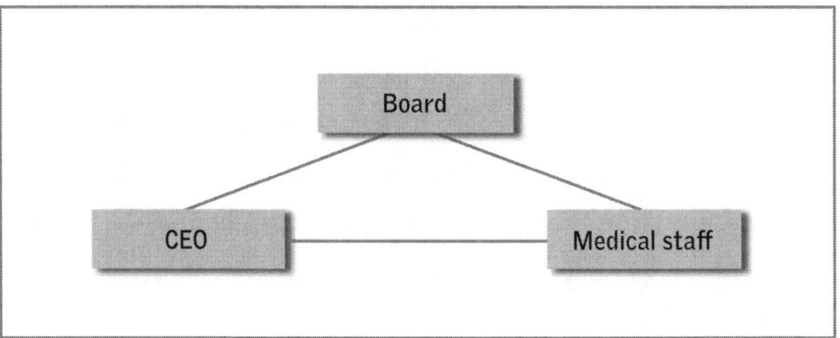


A department chair's jobs of advocating for the medical staff and fulfilling delegated responsibilities are not always at odds. When a department chair is advocating for patient care or on behalf of medical staff members, he or she is fulfilling the board-delegated responsibility to ensure the quality of medical care. You won't find this balancing act outlined in medical staff bylaws, accreditation requirements, or healthcare law, but the model is alive and kicking in your medical staff, and you need to be aware of it.

In addition to advocating for the medical staff, a department chair must partner with the medical staff and ensure that the medical staff is an effective partner for management and the board. Because physicians are accountable to the hospital, yet must partner with the hospital to ensure organizational success, the department chair plays a critical role in fostering these relationships, working to secure open communication, and balancing the interests of all parties. When conflicts arise between the medical staff and management/board, the department chair must use good judgment to help resolve the issue.

Before assuming your role as department chair, you must decide for whom on your medical staff you will advocate. All physicians within your department? A subset of physicians? The entire medical staff? Advocacy is complicated because physicians' interests are not all in alignment. As a department chair you need to be a committed statesperson, not simply act in your self-interest.

  

## The Medical Staff's Major Functions

Most medical staffs, unless they are quite small, have a credentials committee responsible for credentialing and a medical staff quality committee responsible for peer review. We'll come back to responsibilities for credentialing and peer review shortly, but for now we'll discuss the relationship of the department chair to each of these committees.

The department chair reports and is accountable to the credentials committee. When a department chair reviews the file of a medical staff applicant and makes a recommendation, he or she makes that recommendation to the credentials committee. Keep in mind that the department chair is not responsible for making a final decision—only for making a recommendation for the credentials committee to consider when making its recommendation to the MEC regarding medical staff appointment. The same holds true when a department chair recommends criteria for membership with privileges. The credentials committee takes the recommended criteria into consideration and makes a recommendation to the MEC, which in turn makes its own decision.

In terms of peer review, the department chair often does the first peer review or chart review to evaluate a physician's performance. The chair's work measuring performance is accountable to the quality committee (if you have one for your medical staff) or peer review committee, which in turn is accountable to the MEC.

  

If your medical staff is small enough that you don't have a credentials committee or a medical staff quality committee, the department chair is directly accountable to the MEC for these functions. If you are Joint Commission–accredited, keep in mind that neither The Joint Commission nor any other accreditor requires you to have a credentials committee or a medical staff quality committee. If you have one, it's because you've decided it's the best way to get the work of the medical staff done.

## Roles of the Department Chair

1. Recommend criteria for privileges for all specialties assigned to the department—note the word "recommend." The department does not own privilege criteria. The department chair may want his or her department to discuss criteria and make a recommendation, but that's all it is: a recommendation. The recommended criteria go to the credentials committee, which in turn recommends criteria to the board. Because of the department chair's subject matter expertise, though, he or she is most often best positioned to make recommendations, and since the committees rely on this expertise, they look to the department chair to fulfill this responsibility. A challenge arises when criteria recommendations spark cross-specialty disputes. We will address this challenge when we discuss credentialing and privileging in detail.

  

2. Review credentials files and recommend action on all initial appointments and reappointments for department practitioners. This is done by carefully reviewing a practitioner's credentials file and recommending the appropriate action.

3. Review and recommend action on all requests for privileges from department practitioners. Practitioners may have already gone through the application or reappointment process and are now requesting additional privileges. Such requests will come through the department chair for review.

4. Participate in peer review (i.e., measurement) consistent with the medical staff's peer review process. Your medical staff has a process for measuring physician performance and providing feedback. The department chair's role in this process will vary. In some medical staffs, the department chair does all of the initial chart review. In others, he or she is the final arbiter of the chart review. In still others, the chair may have a peer review committee within the department. A medical staff may even remove individualized chart review within a department and instead opt for a centralized peer review committee.

5. Oversee and improve (i.e., manage) the quality of care and professional conduct of individuals granted privileges

  

and assigned to that department. The department chair is responsible for the performance of everyone in his or her department. In short, all physicians within the department are accountable to the department chair for their quality of care and professional conduct in the organization. Many physicians, however, don't understand this accountability, leaving department chairs with an uphill battle. The first step for the department chair is to own this management role. The second is to lead in a way that secures buy-in from physicians to hold themselves accountable.

6. Review and, when appropriate, take action on any reports referred to the chair from other medical staff and hospital committees. Committees will say, "We need the department chair to weigh in on our anticoagulant regimen" or, "We need the chair's input on our block booking policy." The department chair may incorporate input from the medical staff or from his or her department when conducting such reviews, but at the end of the day it's his or her job to make the appropriate recommendations or take the appropriate actions.

7. Perform any relevant activities assigned by the MEC or management (e.g., develop new policies, investigate new technology, evaluate a department-specific matter, etc.). These activities require the department chair's

  

expertise to be effective. A department chair may carry out these functions or delegate them to others and hold them accountable to complete the task timely and effectively.

8. Represent the interests and needs of the department to other departments and members of the management team. This responsibility ties into the department chair's advocacy role. He or she represents the department to other departments and works to ensure effective collaboration with those departments and with the management team.

9. Orient new members to the department. The department chair plays a critical role in orienting new members and communicating the department's expectations. The chair should show new members the ropes, outline performance expectations, and explain how new members will be held accountable. The orientation should go beyond mundane issues like where new members should park, dictating cases, etc.

10. Collaborate with nursing, management, and medical staff leadership on all matters pertaining to the department and the patient care its members provide. We delve into this topic in another section of this handbook.

  

CHAPTER 2

# The Power of the Pyramid: How to Achieve Great Practitioner Performance

It is not unusual to hear from a department chair that he or she has held the leadership role for many years yet never received the training needed to feel comfortable carrying out department chair responsibilities. The purpose of this chapter is to review the power of the pyramid and explain how this model can help medical staff organizations achieve great practitioner performance. This model was created by the late Howard Kirz for the American College of Physician Executives (ACPE) and is focused on the objective of improving physician performance by decreasing conflict and helping each physician be the best that he or she can be.

In the past, hospitals attempted to improve performance by identifying low outliers. In other words, they attempted to identify the "bad apples" by conducting case review and trying to find any medical errors, omissions, and poor patient outcomes. The problem with this approach is that as soon as you identify and rid the organization of a bad apple, another one soon comes along. Figure 2.1 represents a normative bell-shaped performance curve, in which the shared area represents the bad apples.

Figure 2.1

**BAD APPLE PERFORMANCE CURVE**

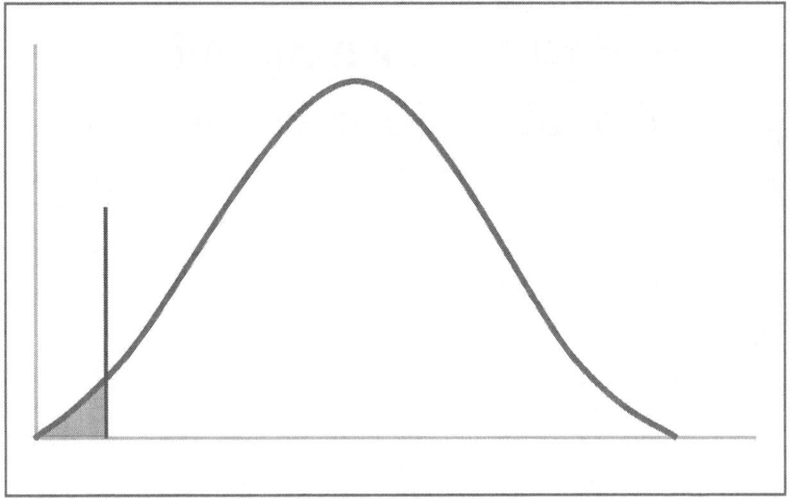

A more effective and positive approach is to follow a model that strives to move the performance of the entire medical staff to the right of the curve and improve the performance of the organization as a whole. Take a look at Figure 2.2. You will notice that the area around the "bad apple" no longer exists. It is no longer under any part of the curve, and every physician—even the strongest-performing members of the team—has the opportunity to improve.

In contrast with the bad-apple approach is the performance improvement pyramid model. The idea behind this model is that if an organization focuses on the foundation layers of the pyramid, there is little chance that performance issues will rise to the top of

  

Figure 2.2 THE BAD APPLE THEORY VS. PERFORMANCE IMPROVEMENT

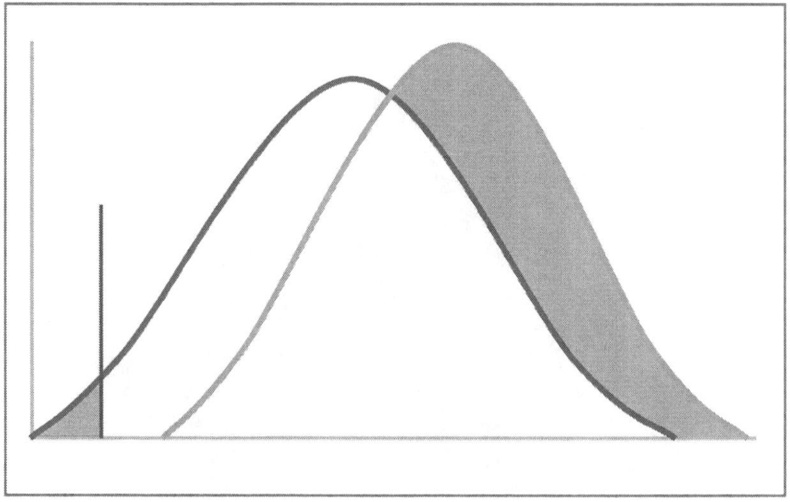

the pyramid and result in corrective action. Figure 2.3 represents the performance improvement pyramid.

Department chairs have the difficult role of maintaining an economic and political relationship with everyone in their clinical department. Understandably, department chairs never want to be forced to take corrective action against any physician, particularly if the physician is an employer, employee, or fierce competitor. Doing so introduces conflicts of interest and could result in political fallout that requires a huge amount of cleanup. To avoid these challenges, follow the pyramid, focus on the foundation layers, and learn to implement the layers effectively.

  

Figure 2.3 **THE PERFORMANCE IMPROVEMENT PYRAMID**

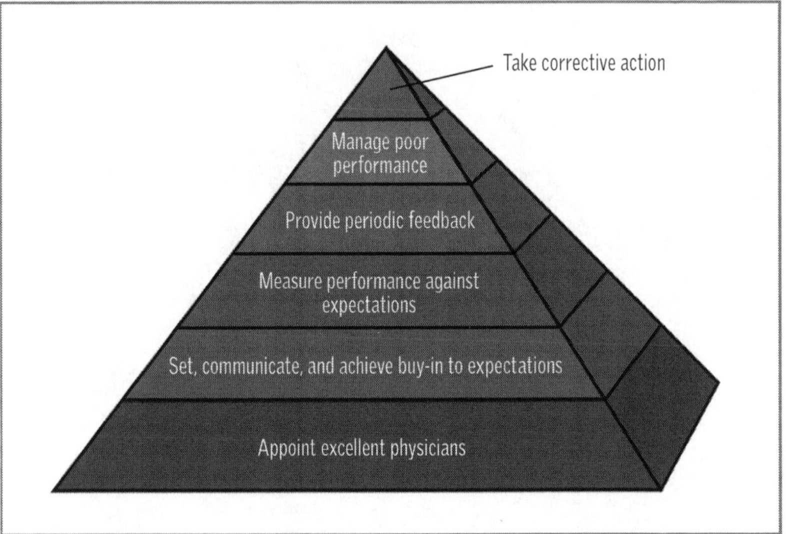


## Appoint Excellent Physicians

Strong physician performance begins with credentialing and privileging. The very best way to address any performance issue is at the door, either at appointment or reappointment. Department chairs should sit down with applicants and review what's expected of them, both as members of the medical staff and members of the clinical department. At reappointment, department chairs should meet with problematic practitioners who are struggling with performance issues, review performance expectations, and gauge practitioners' willingness to commit to meeting those expectations.

Remember, once the physician gets in the door (i.e., is appointed or reappointed), the problem is the department chair's to manage for up to the next two years. To be as proactive as possible, department chairs should address performance issues at this layer of the pyramid. Use the organization's eligibility criteria for both membership and privileges as a guide. Because the department chair recommends eligibility criteria to the credentials committee, the medical executive committee (MEC), and the governing board, it's critically important for the chair to set the bar at a level that he or she feels comfortable implementing and enforcing. Remember that when the department chair helps to address the policies and procedures surrounding credentialing and privileging, he or she must consider the behavioral issues that should be addressed at this layer of the pyramid.

## Set, Communicate, and Achieve Buy-In to Expectations

The next layer of the pyramid—setting, communicating, and achieving buy-in to expectations—is critically important, and one that medical staffs don't always do well. Department chairs should strive to articulate written expectations when interviewing an applicant at appointment, at reappointment, and when performance issues arise. For instance, if the department chair has a team member who struggles with medical records, the chair will be better able to address and resolve that issue if he or she has clearly articulated expectations around medical records and explained the financial and safety impact of incomplete medical records. Put these expectations in writing; as you do, have department members sign off on the expectations and address any concerns, differences of opinion, or lack of buy-in.

Don't forget that performance expectations go beyond technical expectations—they include multiple performance dimensions. Create a framework defining what it means to be a good practitioner in your clinical department and on the medical staff.

You might base your framework on the ACPE and Greeley expectations:

- Technical quality of care
- Quality of service
- Patient safety/patient rights
- Resource utilization
- Peer and coworker relationships
- Citizenship

  

Or, you might choose the Accreditation Council for Graduate Medical Education (ACGME) and The Joint Commission's dimensions of physician performance, which include:

- Patient care
- Medical/clinical knowledge
- Practice-based learning and improvement
- Interpersonal and communication skills
- Professionalism
- Systems-based practice

There is a great deal of overlap between the ACPE and the ACGME performance expectations. See Figure 2.4.

It is essential that you choose a framework to define what it means to be a good practitioner in your clinical department and on the medical staff. Department chairs should accept responsibility for recommending a framework to the quality committee and the credentials committee. These committees will then recommend a framework to the MEC and the governing board.

  

Figure 2.4

### Comparison of The Joint Commission's general physician competencies with the physician pyramid dimensions

| Joint Commission | Patient care | Medical knowledge | Practice based learning | Interpersonal/ communication skills | Professionalism | Systems based practices |
|---|---|---|---|---|---|---|
| Pyramid | | | | | | |
| Technical quality | X | X | X | | | |
| Service quality | X | | | X | | X |
| Patient safety/rights | X | | X | | X | X |
| Resource use | X | X | X | | | X |
| Relationships | | | | X | X | |
| Citizenship | | | | | X | X |

  

## Measure Performance Against Expectations

Once you set, articulate, and achieve buy-in to expectations, you want to measure performance against expectations. Department chairs should recommend to the quality committee performance metrics with two targets: one to recognize excellence, and the other to recognize good performance and separate it from performance that needs follow-up. This will be part of a practitioner's feedback report, or ongoing professional practice evaluation, which is part of the department chair's responsibilities. We'll talk more about this role later in the handbook. The key point to remember is that the department chair should set performance benchmarks and metrics in which to measure and improve physician performance.

## Provide Periodic Feedback

The quality committee, with oversight from the MEC, should provide a feedback report to physicians every six to eight months. The department chair should review these reports with individual department practitioners. Providing physicians with these reports and engaging them in a discussion about the data gives them the opportunity to correct their clinical performance.

Department chairs should be prepared for physicians to push back and say the data is imperfect. Remind physicians that their profession is both art and science. Although it's easy to measure objective data for a science, it's much harder to measure performance data for an art. If physicians fail to buy into expectations, if they can't measure up to your expectations through metrics, or if they won't respond constructively to feedback, you need to move to the next level of the pyramid to manage poor performance.

## Manage Poor Performance

Managing poor performance is a pyramid within a pyramid, composed of the following five layers:

1. **Collegial intervention**

   If an issue arises—whether it's related to conduct, noncompliance with core measures, or noncompliance with the medical records policy—the department chair should first engage in a collegial dialogue with the practitioner and help him or her understand why the performance measure or expectation in question is important. Help the physician understand how the measure or expectation ties into overall performance assessment. Ideally, you'll get the physician to document his or her willingness to comply and/or work with the department chair toward improvement. The department chair should also sign that document. If the physician fails to improve his or her performance following this discussion, the organization must move to the next step of creating a voluntary action plan.

  

2. **Voluntary action plan**

A physician may balk at creating an action plan, in which case the department chair must tell him or her, "If you're unwilling to create and follow a voluntary action plan, we'll have to develop a mandatory action plan, and that is far less collegial." Typically most physicians will want to maintain as much autonomy and freedom as possible and will opt for the voluntary action plan.

Within a voluntary action plan, address improvement that is measurable and include both positive and negative consequences for compliance with the plan. Also include time frames. For instance, make it clear that if the physician complies with the voluntary improvement plan within three months, the organization will go back to purely collegial intervention.

3. **Mandatory action plan**

If the voluntary action plan is unsuccessful, the next layer of the pyramid is a mandatory action plan. The department chair should draft this improvement plan with oversight by the MEC and the quality committee. Ensure the action plan includes measurable data—for example, require the physician to cut medical records deficiencies or validated complaints in half. Have the physician sign the plan, sign it yourself, and create a time frame for compliance. For example, consider including a statement that says if the physician complies with the mandatory improvement plan for six to 12 months, he or she will then move to a voluntary improvement plan for three months; if able to successfully comply with the voluntary plan for three months, he or she will move down the pyramid to purely collegial intervention.

4. **Final warning**

   Finally, the upper layer of the pyramid is what we call the "doc in the box" letter or final warning. At this stage, the organization (department chair, MEC, and governing board) must state exactly what the physician must do to avoid corrective action. Document opportunities for improvement, specific performance metrics, and time frames. Again, consider including positive consequences even in a final warning, stating that if the physician complies with the parameters set out in the warning, he or she can go back to a mandatory action plan, back to a voluntary action plan, and back to purely collegial intervention.

5. **Take corrective action**

   Should the final warning fail to result in performance improvement, the organization must move into corrective action. Corrective action is any step the organization takes that decreases a physician's current clinical privileges or political membership rights on the medical staff. Again, the organization should do everything possible to focus on the foundation layers of the pyramid, taking preventive and proactive actions, and thus avoid having to take corrective action. Understand that if you absolutely must "splash the cold water in someone's face" because the person can't or won't take steps to improve performance, you can issue a precautionary suspension for up to 14 days without having to offer due process rights and up to 30 days without having to make a report to the National Practitioner Data Bank.

Note: A step is added to the performance pyramid when dealing with contracted members of the medical staff in your clinical department. Service agreements and professional or exclusive contracts should include performance metrics, targets, and positive and negative consequences of complying with these expectations. Should a performance issue arise, not only do the department chair, the MEC, and the governing board have authority, but whomever signs their contract also has legally binding authority to hold the physician accountable.

  

CHAPTER 3

# The Department Chair's Role in Credentialing and Privileging

In this chapter we discuss the department chair's role in credentialing and privileging in more detail. Again, we reference the organizational chart to illustrate the department chair's responsibility to make recommendations to the credentials committee, which then makes medical staff membership and privileging recommendations to the medical executive committee (MEC). See Figure 3.1 below.

Figure 3.1 THE MEDICAL STAFF'S MAJOR FUNCTIONS

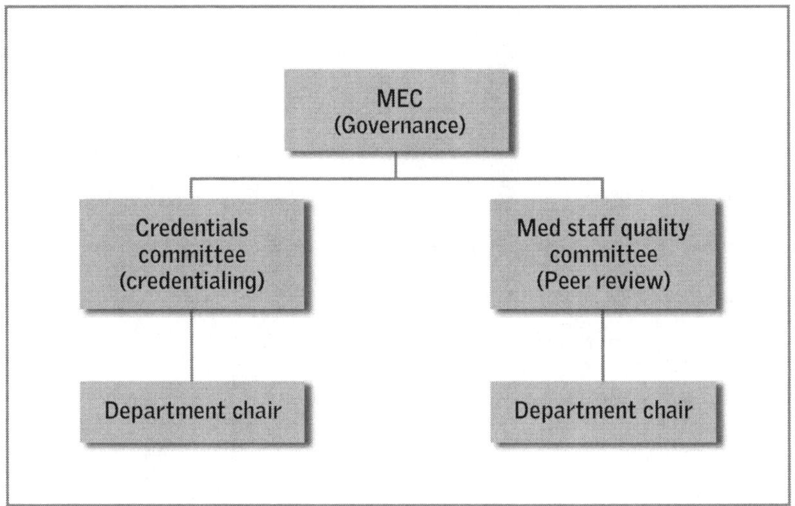


  

Before we delve into the department chair's specific role, it's important to review the definitions of credentialing and privileging because many people confuse the two.

## What Is Credentialing?

The primary goal of credentialing is verifying a physician's credentials to practice medicine—license, training, and malpractice insurance. When credentialing practitioners, you are attempting to determine whether they are who they claim to be. Whenever feasible, information should be verified from the original or primary source of the credential (e.g., the institution that issued the document). Some sources, like the AMA Masterfile, are deemed as though they were a primary source because they went to the primary source, verified, and can vouch for the validity of the data.

Credentialing may appear simple at first, but a lot of careful work has to be done to ensure the integrity of the information collected through the verification process. There are unscrupulous people out there who are masquerading as physicians; there are physicians who are trained but represent themselves to be other than who or what they really are. The credentialing process aims to sniff these people out and ensure your organization does not allow them access to your patients.

  

## What Is Privileging?

After the organization verifies a practitioner's credentials through the credentialing process, the next step is privileging that practitioner. Privileging aims to determine what a practitioner is competent to do within the institution. Data gathered through the privileging process allows the organization to match the privileges it grants to the physician with his or her current competence.

Demonstrating current competence is the single most challenging aspect of credentialing and privileging today. At one point, a physician was considered competent simply by failing to demonstrate incompetence—a philosophy that could also be phrased as "no news is good news." The bar has since been raised. In fact, The Joint Commission now requires hospitals to collect evidence of demonstrated current competence to ensure that privileging is an objective, evidence-based process.

All organizations, whether beholden to Joint Commission standards or not, should aim to collect evidence of physician competence to ensure the organization provides exceptional patient care. Regulatory compliance is simply a byproduct.

## Four Steps in the Credentialing and Privileging Process

Although complex, the credentialing and privileging process can be broken down into four steps:

  

**Step 1:** Establish policies and rules. In this step, the department chairs must work with the MEC and credentials committee (ultimately approved by the governing board). The organization must determine what constitutes the criteria for membership and privileges, what constitutes a completed application, what references should look like, the process for delineating privileges, who evaluates and makes recommendations, and who has what authority. All of these details must be determined when creating policies, rules, and procedures.

**Step 2:** Collect and summarize information in what will ultimately be the completed application. This is primarily the responsibility of management. The medical staff services department has credentialers who will take a physician's completed application, perform primary source verification, and query whomever they need to—references, the National Practitioner Data Bank, the malpractice carrier, and so on. The medical staff leader also has a role in this step, which we will come back to when we deal with the department chair's role in calling references.

**Step 3:** Evaluate and recommend. We now have a completed application, and somebody must evaluate it and make a recommendation. This is a primary and crucial role of the department chair. Your job is to review the application—whether it's for initial appointment, reappointment, or an application for new privileges or technology. You must evaluate the application using all of your clinical expertise, drawing on subject matter experts and their input if necessary. At the end of the day, it is a Joint Commission requirement that the department chair makes a recommendation regarding the practitioner's membership, what category of the medical staff he or she will be in, and privileges. Once your recommendation is made, it will go to the credentials committee, which will give its own recommendation, and the MEC, which will also give a recommendation.

**Step 4:** Grant or deny. Somebody must decide whether to grant or deny (or perhaps modify) the request for membership and privileges. This is often the responsibility of the governing board or its appointed agent.

## Department Chair Credentialing Responsibilities

Let's look at the department chair's credentialing responsibilities in detail:

Recommend criteria for privileges for all specialties assigned to the department. As a chair, this is your job. You may get input from subject matter experts if you're in medicine or surgery and dealing with a specialty outside of your personal expertise, but at the end of the day, it is your recommendation to make. Again, note the emphasis on the word "recommend." We'll come back later to examine what happens when there is a privileging dispute.

Review credentials files and recommend action on all initial appointments and reappointments for practitioners assigned to the department. This is the third step in the credentialing process outlined previously, and it is one of the department chair's most important responsibilities.

Review and recommend action on all requests for privileges from department practitioners. When a practitioner already possesses a set of privileges and requests additional privileges, your job is to review the request and recommend the appropriate action: approve the request, modify it, deny it, or say the practitioner is ineligible to apply due to not meeting criteria. (We'll come back to this last option later.)

Assist the hospital in determining if and how new technology should be adopted. The influx of new technology into hospitals is only going to accelerate. However, does this mean that you have to use a piece of new technology simply because it's there, or because a physician obtained training in it and requested additional privileges to use it? No. The first question that your job requires you to ask is whether a given service will be provided by the hospital, and whether new technology should be incorporated by the hospital.

  

It's also part of your job to keep abreast of new technology and alert the hospital if a given technology is something it may encounter in the near future.

Be available to render judgments on whether a specific procedure, piece of equipment, or new technique requires the granting of additional privileges or the extension of existing knowledge and skills. This is a 24/7 job with many shades of gray involved. Inevitably, somebody is going to book a case in the OR or in the interventional radiology suite that makes use of a new piece of equipment, and someone else is going to say, "Wait a minute, do you have privileges to do this?" This person may then have to call someone to rule on the issue. Ultimately, you're the one to make this ruling. You have to learn to distinguish between cases in which physicians are making use of their existing body of knowledge and skills, and cases in which additional training, experience, and evidence of current competence may be required. If you're unsure about any given case, your fallback position should be to say "no." You are perfectly authorized to do so. Don't feel like you have to approve a new piece of equipment or technology just because a practitioner is requesting it or has already scheduled a case with it. You have the authority to request that more research be done first.

Collaborate with practitioners within your department and other departments on developing criteria for cross-specialty privileges. Others may replace the term "cross-specialty privileges" with the term "turf battles." Do this professionally—this is not about "turf." In fact, if you look up "turf" in Webster's dictionary, the fourth or fifth definition is "something groups of adolescent boys fight over." That's not what being a doctor is about. Yes, there's a pressure to find other sources of revenue, and there are lots of reasons for privileging disputes, but remember that these are disagreements among professionals, not teenage boys. This issue goes back to the question of advocacy discussed in Chapter 1. It's appropriate to advocate for your department, but it's also important to act as a mediator and say, "We need to be thoughtful about this and make it fair and balanced to everybody." The goal, again, is physician success, not just for your department but for other departments; the goal is also balance, hospital success, and good patient care. That's the spirit in which you should play a role when cross-specialty privileging disputes occur.

Recommend and oversee the process of establishing practitioner competency for all newly granted privileges—focused professional practice evaluation, or FPPE. FPPE is a term introduced by The Joint Commission in 2007, and it refers to two different activities: one is when a longtime member of your medical staff applies for privileges they haven't been granted in your organization before, and the other is when a new practitioner joins your medical staff. FPPE is the piece you own as a department chair.

When a practitioner joins the medical staff, how do you know how good he or she is? You've got references, you may have letters from a training program, but you don't have any knowledge about how the person actually practices. Your job is to figure out how to assess the physician's practice. Do you assess it prospectively? Retrospectively? Through proctoring? Through looking at performance data? You must recommend the appropriate process to evaluate the physician's competence for the requested privileges and then ensure those processes are done well. You may not take part in the actual process—maybe your section chief or some other subject matter expert will be doing the proctoring—but your job is to oversee and to make sure it's done in a timely and effective manner.

### *Critical function of evaluating a credentials file*

Think of your hand on a smooth surface. When you're evaluating a credentials file, that's what it should be like, because most applications are smooth and have no red flags. When you review this file, you are usually following after the medical staff professional or credentialer who put the file together—meaning you're the first physician to look at it and assess for red flags. A good credentialer or medical staff professional will draw your attention to potential issues, including:

- Gaps in training or practice
- Previous corrective action
- Professional competence or conduct issues

- Incomplete or inaccurate information provided on the application
- Unusual requests based on background or training
- Unusual background or training
- Multiple changes in practice sites
- That "funny feeling" inside

Don't just take the credentialer's word for it, though. Take the time to go through the file, look at whatever has been highlighted for you, and then look at the other information. Look for any of the red flags listed above. If you find one—and remember, at this point it's just a "bump," not an actual problem—your job is to drill down into that bump and determine whether something is a concern. Remember, the whole exercise of credentialing and privileging is to predict, as accurately as possible, a practitioner's performance over the next few years within your organization. It's not an exact science, but you want to get it as right as you can—patients are counting on you.

If you find a red flag in a practitioner's file, it doesn't mean the person is a bad doctor. Rather, it means you need to dig deeper. Why did that gap happen? Why does the person have so many malpractice cases? Maybe you need to pull the practitioner's medical records. If the person had a professional action at another hospital, what happened? You are entitled to ask for that additional information—that's known as placing the burden on the applicant. If you as a department chair feel you don't have enough data to make an informed decision regarding approval or denial, ask for more information. Let the credentials committee or the medical staff office know what you require, then let them go out and gather it. Don't make a recommendation until you have all the information you need.

### *How to evaluate a credentials file*

When evaluating the credentials files, don't look only at gaps that might be fairly obvious, but also look at references. How do you evaluate references? Physicians often say, "No one will tell the truth in references." They'll claim that they're worthless, that they just serve to whitewash problems, or that they won't reveal a problem for fear of being sued. All of that is true. However, very often there will be hints in a reference—perhaps something is left blank, or a list of ratings contains one "good" rating when everything else is listed as "excellent." These are red flags, and they require you to read between the lines. If you ever get a reference that says, "I'd be happy to share additional information with you," that's saying, "Please call me!"

Calling references is a great tool. You don't have time to call every reference for every applicant, but you should pick up the phone for any applicant who has a "bump" or who gives you that uneasy feeling. What if, when you call, someone asks, "Is this on the record or off the record?" Your job is to say it's on the record. If the next answer is, "Then I can't tell you anything," what do you do? You document it. Thank the reference, hang up the phone, and document all the information you have: the date and time, your name and the name of who you called, the question of whether the call was on or off the record, and the reference's refusal to speak further. Sign the document. What do you have? A bump.

When a "bump" is identified, drill down to resolve the concern to your satisfaction.

Before investigating further, you may request the physician applicant to submit a special release that states he or she will not sue in response to any information the investigation may turn up. It is important that you document all steps in this process to create a paper trail should the investigation result in an adverse credentialing or privileging decision.

Once the "bumps" are identified, it's time for the department chair to risk stratify. This is what the credentials committee and the MEC need from you. The credentials committee and MEC rely on the department chair as the subject matter expert in the specialty area to rate the application. A clean application with no red flags is an R-1, or risk level one. Does an application have a minor bump that you've drilled down into and resolved yourself? That's an R-2. Does an application have a large bump or multiple bumps that require more attention and investigation? That's an R-3. Spend your time drilling down into an R-3 application. Remember to explain why an application is rated an R-2 or R-3 so that everyone who sees the application understands the rating. The credentials committee, the MEC, and the governing board will almost always agree with the department chair's recommendation and they depend on the chair to act in the best interests of the organization and patients. As department chair, that's a weighty responsibility. Take it seriously and do it well.

  

CHAPTER 4

# The Department Chair's Role in Peer Review, Quality, and Patient Safety

This chapter discusses the department chair's key roles and functions related to overseeing peer review, quality, and patient safety. The vast majority of medical staff bylaws specify that the department chair is responsible for overseeing and improving quality of care and conduct on behalf of the medical executive committee (MEC) and the governing board.

As illustrated in Figure 3.1, the MEC is the governing structure of the organized medical staff. The MEC delegates, per its board-delegated authority, credentialing and privileging to the credentials committee. The department chair makes his or her recommendations directly to the credentials committee about criteria and appointment for membership and privileges.

The MEC delegates the role of overseeing and approving the quality aspects of the organized medical staff to the quality or peer review committee. The department chair also plays a key role in partnering with the quality and/or peer review committee to recommend performance metrics and targets, and overseeing peer

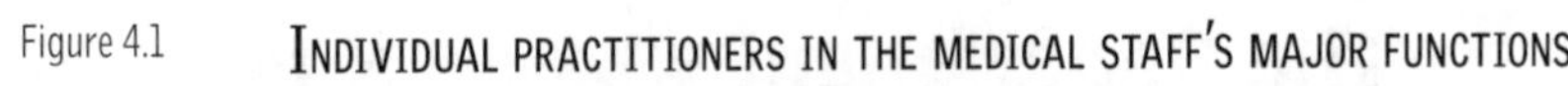

Figure 4.1 INDIVIDUAL PRACTITIONERS IN THE MEDICAL STAFF'S MAJOR FUNCTIONS

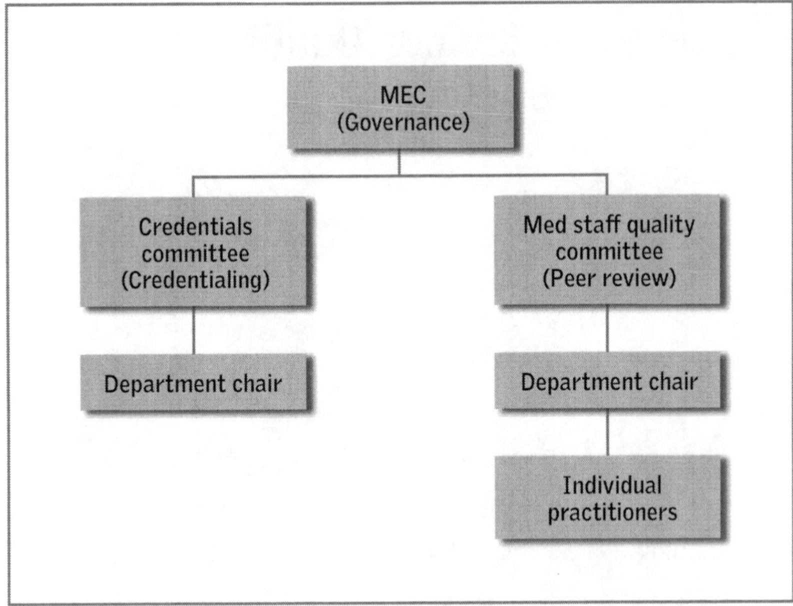


review on behalf of his or her clinical department. The department chair may also be responsible for improvement initiatives as a result of peer review that is performed both in the clinical department and in a centralized peer review committee (if the organization has such a committee). Remember that individual practitioners within the chair's department or service are directly accountable to the chair for the quality of care and services that they provide. See Figure 4.1.

  

## Redefining Peer Review

The traditional definition of peer review is the evaluation of patient charts to determine the quality of care provided by an individual physician. This quality assurance approach of reviewing charts for negative outliers is not an effective model for improving performance and conduct.

The contemporary definition of peer review is the evaluation of an individual physician's professional performance for all relevant performance dimensions—not just technical performance—using multiple sources of performance data.

This contemporary definition takes into account several factors. First, peer review should include a review of aggregate data. The review should consider a broader framework of physician performance, not just how well the physician cuts and sews or diagnoses and treats. This broader definition encourages reviewers to look for opportunities to improve performance, not just opportunities to identify negative outliers.

  

## Performance Dimensions

The department chair is responsible for defining and analyzing several performance dimensions. See Figure 4.2 below.

Figure 4.2 PERFORMANCE DIMENSIONS FOR WHICH DEPARTMENT CHAIRS ARE RESPONSIBLE

- Technical
- Service
- Patient safety/rights
- Utilization
- Peer & coworker relations
- Citizenship
- Patient care
- Medical/clinical knowledge
- Practice-based learning & improvement
- Interpersonal & communication skills
- Professionalism
- Systems-based practices

American College of Physician Executives/The Greeley Company's dimensions of performance include:

- Technical
- Service
- Patient safety/patient rights
- Utilization

  

- Peer and coworker relations
- Citizenship

Accreditation Council for Graduate Medical Education/The Joint Commission's general competencies include:

- Patient care
- Medical/clinical knowledge
- Practice-based learning and improvement
- Interpersonal and communication skills
- Professionalism
- Systems-based practice

The department chair creates the performance framework and determines performance measurements for practitioners within his or her department. The chair is responsible for overseeing and improving all of these chosen dimensions. The framework developed by the chair will be used to conduct ongoing professional practice evaluation (OPPE), which is a routine measurement of all practitioners granted privileges within the clinical department. OPPE involves performance measurement, evaluation of that measurement, and systematic follow-through.

  

Systematic follow-through refers to the steps taken after the peer review or the quality measurement process identifies opportunities for improvement. Don't just put the results in a drawer. Document those opportunities in the physician feedback report and create an improvement process plan for that physician. The department chair is then accountable to the quality committee, the MEC, and the governing board for ensuring that plan is followed.

## OPPE for Department Chairs

In regard to OPPE, the department chair is responsible for recommending performance indicators and targets to the quality committee and for performing case reviews when requested. Let's discuss these tasks in more detail.

A performance indicator helps determine how well something is working (or not working). For example, a department chair may create an indicator to measure how well the organization's medical records system and individual physician performance related to medical records completion is working.

### *Classifying indicators*

There are three categories of indicators: rule, rate, and review. Typically physician leaders are most familiar with review indicators, which require reviewing a specific case to draw conclusions about performance in that case. However, such reviews can be tedious and a waste of time and resources. Reviewing all returns to the operating room, all patient complaints, all unexpected returns to the hospital requires examining hundreds of records—the majority of which are free from problems.

An effective alternative is reviewing aggregate data using rule indicators. Aggregate data allows the organization to take measured action in response to a physician's failure to meet performance metrics rather than acting on a single violation. For example, aggregate data comes in handy when monitoring compliance with medical records completion requirements. The organization may decide not to intervene should a physician violate the requirement up to three times. However, by collecting and analyzing compliance data, the department chair will know when a physician fails to comply with the medical records completion requirement a fourth time. At that point, the department chair may meet with the physician to discuss the importance of medical records and/or send the physician a letter that cites the requirement and provides information about the consequences of noncompliance. If a fifth violation occurs, the department chair may work with the quality committee to create an improvement plan. A sixth violation may escalate the issue to the MEC, and a seventh instance of noncompliance may bring the issue to the governing board and result in corrective action.

Rate indicators have a numerator and denominator. For example, rate indicators for physicians in OB-GYN may include primary C-section rate, episiotomy rates, or the rate of unexpected returns to the OR. To measure rates, the department must first determine targets for both excellent and satisfactory performance.

The use of rate indicators may make it more difficult to accurately assess a physician with low volume. For example, if a physician treats very few patients with a particular condition, it doesn't take many patients to significantly impact his or her rate. On the other hand, if a rule indicator is applied to a low-volume physician, it is not likely that physician will set off a trigger that results in action to improve performance.

As noted above, the department chair's response to performance indicators varies depending on whether that indicator is a rule, rate, or unusual event. If a physician's performance doesn't align with a selected rule, the department chair must provide the physician with immediate feedback and track compliance with that indicator until the physician hits a critical threshold. If using rate indicators, the chair must evaluate the data and create an improvement plan should the physician exceed targets. Lastly, unusual events require the chair to respond immediately.

### *Systematic assessment*

Systematic assessment requires department chairs to review and assess measurement results and help the organization determine whether the performance issue points to a physician competency challenge or a systems challenge. Peer review is about assessing and improving individual performance. Process improvement is about assessing and improving systemic processes. Morbidity and mortality conferences are about educating practitioners about challenging cases. When focused on peer review or OPPE, the department chair must focus on identifying and improving individual—not system—performance issues.

### *Systematic follow-through*

Systematic follow-through is when you act to address trends and issues when needed by creating improvement opportunities and improvement plans, with accountability to whomever is appropriate.

### *Responding to data*

Figure 4.3 is a histogram that illustrates the number of charts that various clinical departments had to review based on aggregating data. The shaded bar represents case review that required review of all unexpected returns to the operating room and emergency department and all medical records violations.

Also illustrated in Figure 4.3 is the reduction in workload achieved by aggregating the data and looking at critical thresholds that met with both rules and rates. The take-home message is to aggregate data whenever possible. Doing so allows the organization to better spend its time and resources.

  

Figure 4.3 COMPARISON OF CHARTS ACTUALLY REVIEWED TO THOSE REVIEWED WITH THE THREE-CATEGORY SYSTEM

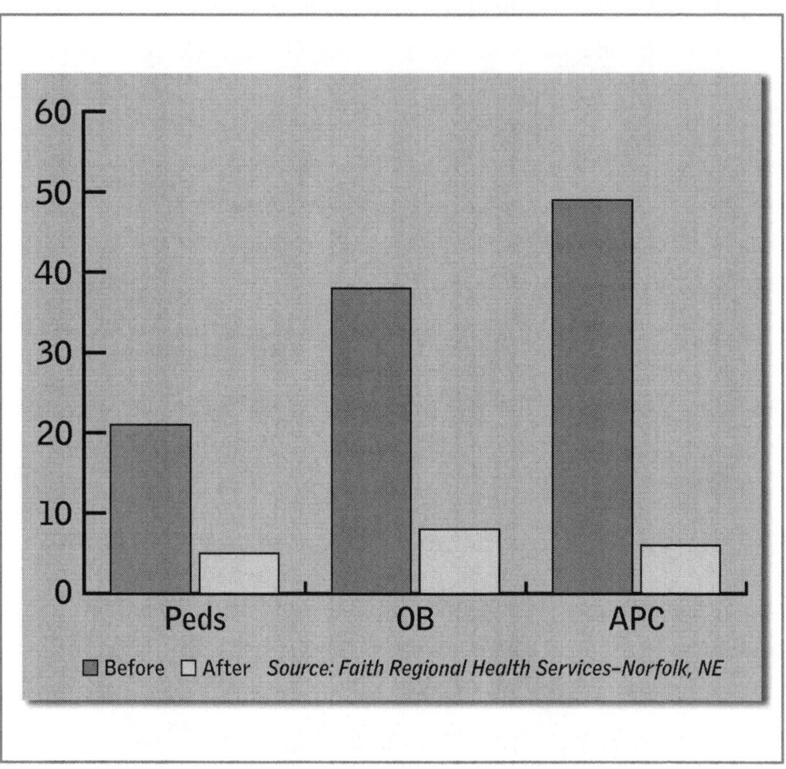


## *Creating indicators*

Once you create your competency framework, you must pick performance measures that tie to each competency. Remember that each performance measure should include two targets, and include that data in the physician feedback report.

  

One of the biggest challenges to creating performance measures for the competencies is determining how to assess the dimensions of physician perception that can only be measured through the eyes and perceptions of others. Take a look at the list of competencies below:

- Technical
- Service
- Patient safety/patient rights
- Utilization
- Peer and coworker relations
- Citizenship
- Patient care
- Medical/clinical knowledge
- Practice-based learning and improvement
- Interpersonal and communication skills
- Professionalism
- Systems-based practice

  

How can the organization accurately measure physician behavior and conduct? Relying on the perceptions of a physician's peers is difficult for physician leaders who traditionally consider a peer as a fellow physician within the same clinical specialty or subspecialty. However, performance measuring requires a physician to accept feedback from outside of his or her specialty or practice, and sometimes outside of his or her profession.

To further illustrate the value of perception data, consider the emergency department physician. Several nonphysicians within the department, including the nurse manager, are privy to that physician's interactions with patients and other practitioners. The perceptions of these nonphysicians are critically important and provide valuable insight into the physician's performance.

### *Additional peer review roles*

Additional peer review roles of the department chair include:

- Contributing to designing and articulating performance expectations
- Cultivating medical staff buy-in to performance expectations
- Cultivating a culture of measurement, continuous performance improvement (PI), and accountability
- Working continuously to improve the peer review process

  

## Frameworks for Healthcare System Performance Improvement

When tackling these challenges, department chairs may wonder whether it is a better use of their time to concentrate on fixing performance or fixing systems. Most organizational challenges can be attributed to systems issues. Therefore, the department chair must concern him- or herself with not only peer review and performance and assessment of individuals, but also with the system around his or her department.

When assessing systems challenges, collaborate with nursing and senior management to address issues that go beyond the performance of individual physicians or practitioners and affect the entire clinical setting. Current frameworks for healthcare system performance measurement provide the department chair with tools that he or she can use to help the MEC, management, and the governing board improve systems.

Total Quality Management is an approach developed by Deming and Dram in the early 20th century. This approach focuses on rapid cycle improvements, or quality circles, with which many physicians are already familiar. Other rapid cycle improvement processes adopted by many organizations are plan, do, check, and act (PDCA) or plan, do, act, assess, and stabilize (PDAAS). PDCA and PDAAS don't require a department meeting before acting and instead allow for on-the-spot improvements. A surgeon can do rapid change cycle management right after an operating procedure by simply asking, "How would we like to do this procedure differently tomorrow?" during a staff debriefing. This is a less formal approach based on teams and specific measurable objectives.

Several hospitals have engaged in the journey toward the Malcolm Baldrige Award, not necessarily to win (because typically only one or two healthcare organizations in the country win every year), but merely to improve their systems' processes. The journey is, frankly, an even greater benefit than the award itself.

ISO 9000, now known as ISO 9001 and ISO 9002, began in Europe and focused on standardizing manufacturing. The standards of ISO, or the International Organization for Standardization, are increasingly being applied to healthcare processes, operations, and procedures. The accreditor DNV (Det Norske Veritas) built standards that align with CMS *Conditions of Participation* and ISO 9000 and 9001 requirements.

Six Sigma aims to reduce errors per million encounters through standardization. Anesthesia standardized its processes by mandating the use of particular anesthesia machines and agreeing to medication labeling standards. As a result, anesthesia achieved Six Sigma or less than three errors per million encounters. Department chairs must question whether allowing 50 practitioners in the department to carry out a procedure 50 different ways actually adds value, or whether it presents an opportunity for unnecessary medical errors.

Lean enterprise was designed and developed by Toyota Enterprise and aims to drive out inefficiency, fat, and waste in the system. It examines processes to see what steps fail to add financial or qualitative value. A classic example in emergency medicine is triage. Many organizations are replacing triage with a medical screening exam. If, through the medical screening exam, the physician determines that the patient does not have an acute emergency medical condition, the patient can then go through proper registration and orientation or be transferred to another facility.

The essential elements of all PI models are as follows:

- Organized
- Teams
- Cycles
- Measurement
- Improvement (not perfection)

To improve organization performance, department chairs must:

- Understand and use the organization's PI methods

  

- Help define clear goals for PI projects
- Participate in organizational PI oversight to prioritize PI efforts
- Participate in organizational PI teams
- Champion PI projects
- Strive for high reliability, not just error reduction

## Ensuring High Reliability

High reliability is the assurance that everyone on your team does the right thing, the first time, every time. Achieving high reliability is a real challenge in a profession that has always honored all practitioners and their right to do it their way every time.

Department chairs can play a key role in determining whether the department will standardize its processes in an effort to reduce error and increase its reliability. To achieve high reliability through a culture of safety, physician leaders must:

- **Understand human error.** Errors are inevitable; the best you can do is to mitigate them, not eliminate them completely.
- **Set expectations for safety.** This involves transparency, reporting errors, and sharing mistakes in a nonretaliatory, nonpunitive environment.

  

- **Provide tools to reduce errors.** Examples include STAR (stop, think, act, and review), three-part acknowledgement of communications, or the adoption of critical, inviolable rules.

- **Ensure accountability.** Do this by communicating expectations and holding physicians accountable should they fail to meet them.

To successfully establish a culture of safety, the department chair must engage physicians not only in his or her department but also within the entire medical staff. How do we engage medical staff in hospital patient safety? First, make it clear that reducing medical errors may require compromising autonomy for the sake of standardization, reliability, and supporting each other in teams of rapid cycle improvements. Also, stress the importance of compliance with safety methods and team leadership so that you as the department chair can play a significant role in reducing errors that may lead to harm and undermine individual performance.

  

CHAPTER 5

# The Department Chair's Role in Managing Poor Performance and Unprofessional Conduct

One of the most vexing and challenging tasks a department chair will face is managing poor performance and unprofessional conduct. As mentioned in Chapter 2, applying the power of the pyramid will help navigate this challenge while keeping in mind the economic and political relationships that exist among physicians in the department.

## Review of the Performance Pyramid Foundation Layers

Remember, as outlined in Chapter 2, the best time to address performance issues is during credentialing and privileging at appointment and reappointment. If not addressed at this stage of the process, the department must own the performance/behavior issue for years to come.

If a physician is struggling with a performance issue, chances are he or she does not understand or does not buy in to performance expectations. The department chair's role is to help the physician understand why the department chair is spending so much time addressing performance issues. Remember that if you can't measure it, you can't manage it, and if you can't manage it, you can't improve it. Therefore, be sure to measure performance against expectations. As W. Edwards Deming said, "In God we trust, all others bring data."

Department chairs must provide periodic feedback, and when a performance issue shows up on a feedback report, they must sit down with the practitioner—a colleague—to review performance data and figure out a way to work together to support improvement for that performance measure.

## Managing Poor Performance

Managing poor performance is a series of carefully crafted, escalating interventions designed to decrease variation from expectations. The most important words here are "carefully crafted," which means the steps must be customized. The department chair cannot conduct an intervention the same way for different practitioners. Escalating interventions means that with each intervention there are escalating consequences as a result of the physician's noncompliance with the performance improvement plan. Don't just go back three or four times and have the same conversation. The first intervention should be different than the second one; the second one should be different from the third one.

  

## Planning the Intervention

Do not go into an intervention without a plan. Plan and practice the intervention. Remember, if a practitioner is a chronic violator or has chronically poor performance, he or she is better at defending him- or herself than the chair may be at conducting an intervention.

### *Who should do the intervention?*

Although the chief of staff or department chair typically conducts the invention, he or she may not always be the best choice. The chief may be a competitor, employer, or employee of the individual. The department chair may opt to assemble a team of individuals to intervene. Perhaps there is a member of the medical staff with a strong relationship with the physician who requires the intervention. That physician may be in the best position to speak frankly and simply say, "Please just cut it out. Get along with other members of the medical staff. We want to maintain your professional standing here."

### *When do you conduct the intervention?*

If it is a critical issue, you may have to deal with it immediately. For example, if a physician throws a tray of instruments in the operating room, you may have to scrub up and deal with it on the spot. Your policies and procedures should document the issues your organization considers egregious and that would result in immediate corrective action. On the other hand, if it is a chronic medical records violation, you may want to wait a week or 10 days to let things cool off before addressing the issue with the physician.

### *Where do you conduct the intervention?*

For an initial intervention, you may go to the physician's office or practice and let the individual sit behind his or her desk. On the other hand, if it's a final warning, you may want to bring the physician into the boardroom to sit with the governing board chair, medical executive committee chair, chief medical officer, CEO, and department chair. This setting makes it clear that the physician is no longer in control and the organization is taking formal action.

### *What should you do in your intervention?*

The steps of an intervention will vary depending on the circumstances. However, there are some common guidelines to keep in mind:

- **Ask the right first question.** Ask the physician why his or her data is different than his or her peers rather than asking why the data is "bad." Discuss with the physician whether the data is valid, measures something that the physician didn't perform, is not attributed correctly, etc. Asking the right first question opens the door to a productive discussion rather than putting the physician on the defensive.

  

- **Listen to the physician's truth.** Before sharing your truth with an individual, listen to theirs. First of all, they may have a legitimate truth—for example, the medical records department may not work, the nurses may be incompetent, or there may be subpar supplies or equipment that they cannot use or that is frustrating to use. The point is, there may be other issues and mitigating circumstances to consider. The physician is more likely to listen to the department chair if first given the opportunity to share his or her viewpoint.

## The Source of Power and Influence

*"Never expect anyone to engage in behavior that serves your values until you have given that person adequate reason to do so."*

—Charles Dwyer

This quote comes from Chuck Dwyer's course "The Source of Power and Influence," which he teaches with the American College of Physician Executives. He summed up his entire life's work with this quote. What is adequate reason for a physician to change his or her behavior? Is it money, professional respect, maintaining his or her standing in the clinical department, or ability to earn a livelihood? Determining this motivating factor can help the department chair prompt the physician to change or be willing to change his or her behavior.

  

## BATNA

Before beginning the intervention, plan your BATNA: Best alternative to a negotiated agreement. Some may call this "Plan B." In other words, if your intervention fails, what would you do?

Consider the example of a disruptive physician who is also the organization's biggest admitter. In fact, imagine the physician generates over $4 million in operating revenue every year for the hospital. Before conducting the intervention with this physician, the department chair says to the board and CEO, "Before I do this intervention, are you willing to lose $4 million in operating revenue next year if this doesn't work out?" The CEO responds that she is not willing to lose the revenue and insists the chair must "fix the problem." The chair appropriately responds that if the physician is unwilling to work with him to fix the problem, the organization may need to take corrective action. The chair then asks for the CEO's assurance in writing that the board and the CEO would accept losing the $4 million in operating revenue if corrective action is necessary.

Make sure that before conducting an intervention, everyone is aware of the potential consequences. If the department chair successfully works with the practitioner to fix the problem, everyone benefits. If unsuccessful, there may have to be a negative consequence for both the practitioner and the hospital.

  

## Goals of Intervention

When planning an intervention, keep in mind the following goals—the response you wish to elicit from the physician:

- Reiteration of the problem or concern
- Acceptance of responsibility for the problem
- Commitment to address the problem
- Commitment to an action plan and goal(s)
- Agreement on how you will both know whether the goal(s) are met
- Commitment to meet again in the near future

An intervention requires that the practitioner with whom the department chair is working acknowledges the concern/competency issue. He or she must accept responsibility. For example, the physician must understand that he or she has not completed medical records in accordance with policy and therefore is unable to effectively communicate patients' conditions to colleagues. Incomplete medical records also means that the physician can't bill for the services delivered and could be found guilty of fraud if he or she does bill for services undocumented in the record. The hospital can't bill for the physician's services, which has a significant financial impact on the organization.

  

After acknowledging the issue and related consequences, the physician must commit to addressing the issue and changing the behavior. The chair and the physician must agree on how change will be measured and agree to meet again in the near future to assess progress toward change.

Before the intervention, determine an acceptable result of the conversation. Would the department chair only accept a response from the physician that exudes gratitude: "Department chair, thank you so much for meeting with me. I deeply appreciate your input. You have changed my life for the better." Or would the chair accept a less gracious response: "I'll follow your darn policy, now please get out of my life." Such a response may suit the chair just fine. Decide a "good enough" outcome before the intervention.

## Practicing the Intervention

The first step in an intervention is to reference your role: "I'm here to talk to you as department chair of emergency medicine [or surgery, or anesthesia]." This step is important because the chair's title brings authority and obligation. Remember, the department chair's obligation under the medical staff bylaws is to enforce all bylaws, rules, regulations, policies, and procedures. Intervening when a performance issue is evident is part of the chair's duty.

The next step is framing the concern in a nonjudgmental way. Frame it as a data issue or performance measurement issue. To return to the example of medical records, the chair may say to the physician, "Your rate of medical records violations is twice that of anyone else on the medical staff." Next, state your intended goal: "I'd like to work with you to cut your rate of medical records violations in half."

Anticipate and prepare for resistance. As mentioned earlier in this chapter, it is often the case that the physician has been dealing with the performance issue in question for quite some time. He or she is likely well versed at defending the behavior and may have more experiences with interventions than the department chair. Preparing for this push-back will help the department chair respond and move the discussion forward.

## Managing Poor Performance

Consider the example of an intervention with a physician with conduct issues. The initial intervention would be a collegial dialogue during which the department chair would ask the physician whether he or she understands the impact of the behavior on patients and the patient care environment. The department chair should reference specific examples of the physician's negative conduct. For instance, "Because you yell at the nurses, they are uncomfortable calling you in the middle of the night, which means you may not have the opportunity to receive critical clinical information that would allow you to make important decisions around your patient's safety and outcomes."

  

Following this collegial conversation, the department chair and physician would ideally sign an agreement that specifies how the chair will support the physician's efforts to correct the deficiency.

If a second intervention is necessary, that conversation should conclude with the signing of an informal action plan. The physician may balk at this less-than-collegial discussion. If so, the department chair may need to threaten to invoke a mandatory action plan. The action plan should include measurable outcomes—data that will determine whether the physician is complying with the plan. The action plan should also spell out the positive consequences for compliance and the negative consequences for noncompliance.

One negative consequence of noncompliance is the necessity of the third intervention to enforce a mandatory action plan. There is little discussion during this intervention. The department chair must command the conversation and make clear that if the physician is unsuccessful in complying with the mandatory action plan, a final warning will follow. On the other hand, if the physician is successful, the next steps are instituting an informal action plan and then collegial interaction.

As noted above, if the physician does not comply with the mandatory action plan, the department chair must issue a final warning. This final warning should state what is required of the physician, the negative consequences if he or she does not comply, and how compliance will be measured. The negative consequence of noncompliance is typically formal corrective action.

## Timing of Meetings

How often you meet with the physician will depend on the circumstances. If you see evidence that the physician is improving, be sure to seize the opportunity to provide positive reinforcement. If the physician is successfully implementing the improvement plan, document the success and put that note in the physician's confidential file. A note to the physician might state, "I want you to know that I appreciate your success at implementing your voluntary action plan, and I would like to acknowledge that your patient and staff complaint rates have dropped significantly. I wish to commend you."

Gradually increase the time between meetings if things are going well or reduce that time if the physician is not improving. Expect and prepare for some backsliding because it is likely to happen. At the first sign of such a backslide, give immediate feedback to provide the physician with constructive support and reinforcement for making a positive change.

## Documentation

Keep in mind the following guidelines regarding documentation of interventions:

  

- Documentation is optional for the initial intervention but required for all others
- Close the intervention by informing the physician that he or she can expect a letter summarizing the discussion
- The physician may provide a written response to the letter, but that doesn't change the content of the letter
- The letter and physician's response both go into the physician's peer review file

It is best practice to document everything. Document that the initial intervention was framed in a positive manner and that the chair expressed appreciation and support for the physician. The chair's signature on such a document indicates that he or she understands his or her obligation as a physician leader.

At the end of the intervention, inform the physician that he or she can expect a letter summarizing the discussion. The chair may opt to write the letter during the intervention, reviewing it with the physician and making any agreed-upon modifications. The chair and physician can both sign the letter at that time.

Although the physician may provide a written response to the letter, his or her rebuttal should not alter the content of the letter. It is helpful to have the physician's perspective when dealing with any peer review or quality issue.

  

As advised previously in this chapter, create an improvement plan that both the department chair and physician sign. A physician with medical records violations may claim that he or she cannot find the files in the medical records department. In such situations, the department chair may include in the improvement plan his or her commitment to try to secure electronic access to the files for all medical staff members. In turn, the physician commits to going to the medical records department every week to sign medical records.

Keep in mind that managing poor performance is really about helping practitioners in the department succeed and securing a safe patient care environment. What can be a difficult and demanding process can also be constructive, collaborative, and beneficial to the practitioner, department, and medical staff as a whole.

  

CHAPTER 6

# The Department Chair's Role in Collaboration and Strategic Planning

The department chair is responsible for advocating for a number of stakeholders—patients, physicians, the department as a whole, and the hospital. The chair ensures patients receive high-quality care, that physicians partner with the organization to deliver this care, and that physicians' abilities to practice are not unfairly limited by hospital actions. In some instances, the chair also advocates for the department when privileging disputes erupt or when under the scrutiny of the quality or peer review committees. The chair also represents the board by effectively carrying out his or her credentialing, privileging, and peer review responsibilities. To traverse this complicated terrain, the chair must learn to balance and fairly represent the interests of all of these stakeholders.

## Balancing Department Chair Roles

It is important to recognize that there is more than one way to effectively get this balance right. However, a department chair will have the most success if he or she approaches this challenge in good faith and with every intention to be fair and impartial. To do this well, keep in mind the following steps:

1. Accept that conflicts of interest will arise. You cannot be in healthcare today and not have conflicts of interest. Focus on handling these conflicts rather than trying to avoid them altogether.

2. Be thoughtful and balanced in fulfilling responsibilities, particularly in representing the interests of the department. Not all physicians in your department will share the same interests. They may compete with one another for revenue and resources. They may also compete with another department for revenue and resources, which could result in a heated privileging dispute. The department chair's job is not to blindly defend the department, but to be thoughtful and balanced.

3. Ensure the medical staff develops and implements clear conflict of interest and confidentiality policies. Conflicts of interest are going to happen. Develop, implement, and adhere to your policies addressing these issues. The policy should require that all members of a deliberative body or in a leadership role must divulge actual or potential conflicts of interest. Based on those disclosed conflicts, the deliberative body then can decide who can and cannot participate in a discussion and/or vote. In regard

  

to confidentiality, department chairs are privy to sensitive information about physicians in the department and about the hospital organization. Treat that information with respect and maintain confidentiality.

4. Be open and transparent when speaking or acting in a leadership role. Make clear what hat you are wearing. For example, the department chair may speak out as a member of the largest OB-GYN group on the medical staff. When doing so, he or she preface comments with the statement, "On behalf of the OB-GYN group ..." When speaking on behalf of the department, he or she should state, "As department chair ..." Further, when sitting with the medical executive committee, the department chair may state that he or she is speaking on behalf of the entire medical staff and acting in the best interest of the hospital and patient care.

5. Understand, contribute to, and support the hospital's strategic plan. The hospital expects department chairs to help make the organization's strategic plan a reality and not just a piece of paper that sits in a drawer and gets dusted off every two years. Department chairs must have input into the strategic planning process, and once approved, the chair's job is to help implement that plan.

6. Seek new solutions to challenges. There is no road map for how to address the thorny issues that will come across

  

a department chair's desk. Be creative and identify new solutions to these challenges. Department chairs who think outside the box develop new approaches that benefit physicians, the hospital, and patients.

## Practices of Successful Department Chairs

The keys to successfully carrying out department chair responsibilities include:

- **Be an outstanding listener.** Seek first to understand, then to be understood. Listen, listen, listen. Get the lay of the land before reacting.

- **Be a statesman.** The department chair can be a key mediator. Remember, politics is the art of the practical. How can you accomplish your goal in a practical and effective way? Conflict is going to occur, but in the presence of good leadership, conflict can be quelled and reasonable heads will prevail. In the absence of good leadership, conflict will escalate. Your job is to make sure that doesn't happen on your watch.

- **Separate "positions" from "interests."** How can the department chair be an effective mediator or negotiator? For example, physicians are going to represent both sides of a privileging dispute. Some will argue, "No practitioner outside this department and without this specific training should have privileging to do this procedure." That's a position. The department chair's job is to acknowledge that position and understand why the practitioner holds that position. Is the physician afraid he or she is going to lose income? Is he or she concerned about patient care? A good listener, a good department chair, will tease out the physician's position.

- **Be an effective mediator.** It's not always the department chair's job to solve the problem, but rather to bring the parties together and help them listen to and understand one another's position.

- **Develop your successor.** Leadership requires knowledge and skills most physicians don't acquire in medical school. It's important that those in leadership positions take an active role in succession planning. Invest in identifying and developing successors for the department.

- **Run a great meeting that others will want to attend.** A great meeting will engage the department and enact real change and improvement. (More on this topic can be found in Chapter 7.)

  

CHAPTER 7

# Effective Department Meetings

Traditionally medical staff department meetings start late, participants arrive unprepared, discussion focuses on routine business and reports, controversial topics are raised and then left unresolved, and the meeting is monopolized by a vocal few. Is it really any wonder department chairs struggle to get physicians to attend these meetings? In this chapter, we review the following rules department chairs can follow to ensure effective, well-attended meetings:

- Plan the agenda
- Start on time
- Limit nonproductive discussion
- Move the agenda
- Assign items for further development

## Agenda

Keep the following guidelines in mind when creating the meeting agenda:

- Schedule a pre-meeting with assistant and advisors. Meet with medical staff services professionals, directors of quality, and perhaps the vice president of medical affairs and/or chief medical officer. Get their input into what issues the department must address.

- Nothing goes on the agenda without the chair's approval and a clear goal for that item. Before adding an item to the agenda, the department chair should ask whether addressing the issue would result in real change or improvement. If not, don't include it. If yes, make clear the goal of the discussion and determine whether it will be a conflict-ridden debate.

- Schedule a pre-meeting with key stakeholders. Don't wait until the meeting to sit down with folks who have real passion or a vested interest in a particularly thorny issue. Begin with seeking first to understand. Listen, mediate, and seek ways to reach a resolution even before the meeting.

- Create a consent agenda for routine business. When reports need to be passed through committee or when a noncontroversial issue needs to come before the department chair, create a consent agenda. In advance of the meeting, send out all materials related to topics on the consent agenda to allow people to review. At the beginning of the meeting, ask whether any attendees would like to pull an issue off the consent agenda to discuss. If so, discuss the issue to the group's satisfaction. If not, make a motion to accept the consent agenda, which will result in those issues being excluded from the proceedings.

- Don't put complex controversial issues on the agenda without adequate preparation. Talk to stakeholders and get needed data. Do your homework and understand what direction the discussion is likely to take. If you know the group will likely not be ready for resolution on a given matter, open the floor for discussion and make clear that resolution is desired but may not be feasible after one discussion.

- Put important items first. There is no need to follow the traditional format of addressing routine or old business first.

- Allot a specific amount of time for each agenda item. Consider the time allotted for the meeting and designate a specific number of minutes to each agenda item. If you stick to that time limit, almost every meeting can be concluded on time.

  

- Prepare materials needed for decision-making in advance so that everyone can review the information prior to the meeting.

## Timing

Many organizations accept what is often referred to as "doc time"—they'll get here when they get here. Remember, people will always arrive late unless the meeting chair establishes that he or she will start the meeting on time, every time. To make this cultural change, the bylaws should define a "quorum" as those present and voting, which must be at least two people. Establishing a quorum and starting the meeting on time makes it clear that the department chair will not allow anyone to hold the meeting hostage. If a physician arrives after the group has discussed an important item, don't go back and rediscuss it or revote. The physician has forfeited the chance to participate by not arriving to the meeting on time.

## Leadership

To establish ownership of the meeting, the department chair should consider the following:

- **Table position.** The department chair should sit at the head of the table or the middle of the table—wherever everyone can see and hear him or her.

  

- **Body language and tone of voice.** Don't underestimate the impact of body language and tone of voice. These are key instruments for establishing leadership and maintaining control of the meeting.

Table position, body language, and tone of voice all communicate the department chair's authority. But keep in mind that the chair should not be authoritarian. He or she is there to lead a group of people, who may not always see eye to eye, through complex discussion and decision-making.

## Discussion and Aims

One of the chair's primary tasks in a meeting is to limit unproductive discussion so as to avoid the "never-ending" meeting that accomplishes nothing. The following tactics can help keep meetings on track:

- Use the meeting to make decisions—avoid using it for emotional expression, endless processing, or a social gathering. There is a time and place for social gathering. There is a time and place for emoting about the things that anger and frustrate department members. If that's the intention of the agenda item, make it so. But when it's time to make a decision, make sure to move the discussion in that direction.

- Solicit input from all participants. In some cases it is appropriate for the department chair to go around the room and solicit input from everyone. Don't allow a vocal few to silence the majority of attendees.

- Establish a bias toward action. Each agenda item should have with it an intended outcome. It must be within the department's sphere of control or sphere of influence—the department must be able to do something as a result of the discussion. For example, members of the department likely care about Medicare reimbursement and healthcare reform, but the department can't make a decision to impact those issues. Don't get bogged down discussing things the department can't change.

## Moving Meetings Along

One of the biggest challenges to managing a meeting is keeping the discussion moving. Keep the following tips in mind to avoid endless meetings that result in little action:

- **Stay on task.** The department chair must be willing to politely interrupt a colleague who has wandered off topic, remind him or her of the discussion at hand, and return to the agenda.

- **Move discussion toward decision.** If discussion is not progressing toward decision, terminate it, and assign one or two interested members to research the agenda item and bring back recommendation.

  

## Consensus and Majority Rule

Are you ruling by consensus or majority? Medical staffs are collegial bodies. We want, by and large, to rule by consensus. However, at the end of the day, majority rule prevents an issue from getting stuck in debate. Working toward consensus is a goal of all leaders and there are some tools for reaching a consensus among department members. Take a look at the following scale that department chairs can use in collecting votes:

+3 We must do this

+2 We should do this

+1 I support this

0 I'm neutral

-1 I don't support this but won't oppose it

-2 We should not do this

-3 We must not do this

Everyone gets a vote. Count the number of +3 votes, +2 votes, etc. Determine where to draw the line for whether consensus is achieved. In most cases, the voting average should be above -2. If above -2, everyone is in support, neutral, or won't oppose it. That's as good a consensus as you're going to get.

The chair must also determine whether he or she will allow the discussion to continue if people feel strongly opposed, or whether the group will move on and let majority rule. By using this type of voting, consensus is reached more often.

  